I0101364

BABA
Goes To Yoga

Written and illustrated
by

Jakki Moore

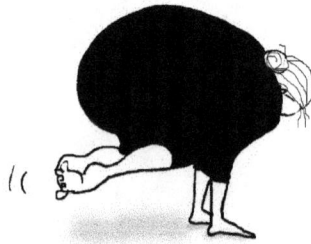

`BABA GOES TO YOGA´
Written and illustrated by Jakki Moore

First published by MoonCat Publications, 2017

Text and drawings copyright © by Jakki Moore

All rights reserved.

No part of this publication may be reproduced, stored in
A retrieval system or transmitted in any form or by any means, electronical,
mechanical, digital, photocopying, scanning
or otherwise, without prior permission of the copyright owner.

ISBN-13: 978-0956410825

ISBN-10: 0956410820

`My mission in life is not merely to survive, but to thrive:

And to do so with some passion, some compassion,

Some humor, and some style.´

-Maya Angelou

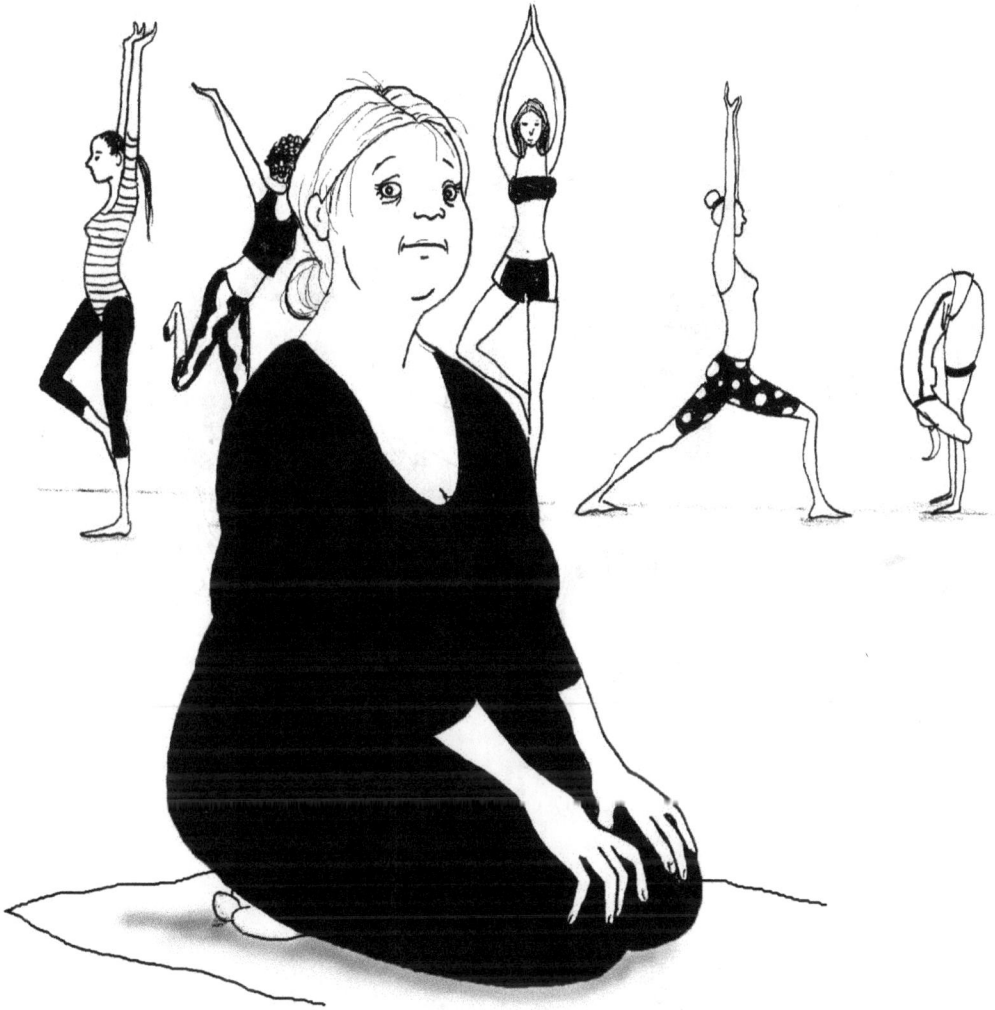

Baba joined a yoga class

And sat on her new mat.

She looked at all the others

Saw none of them were fat.

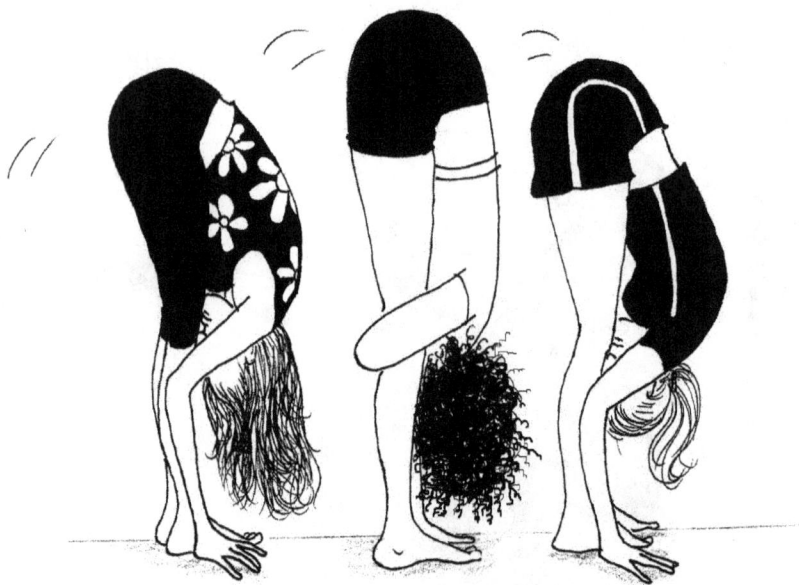

Fit and firm, cool and trendy

Very chic and oh so bendy.

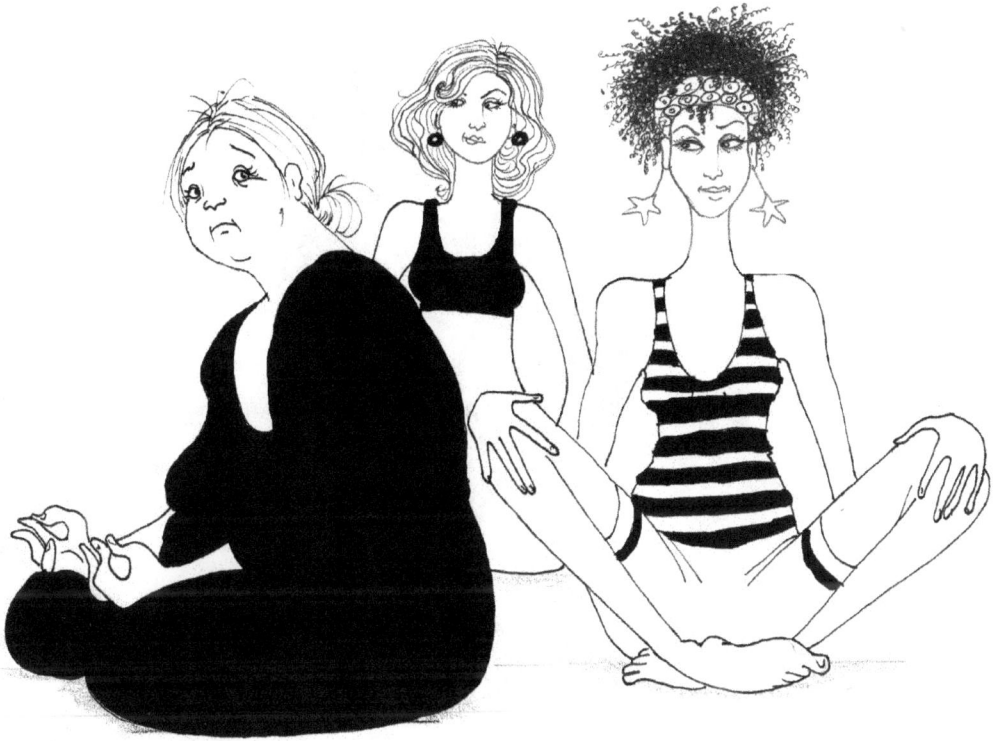

In lycra tops and yoga pants,

They looked at her with heads askance.

Feeling glum and out of place,

`I´ll quit,´she thought, `I might lose face.´

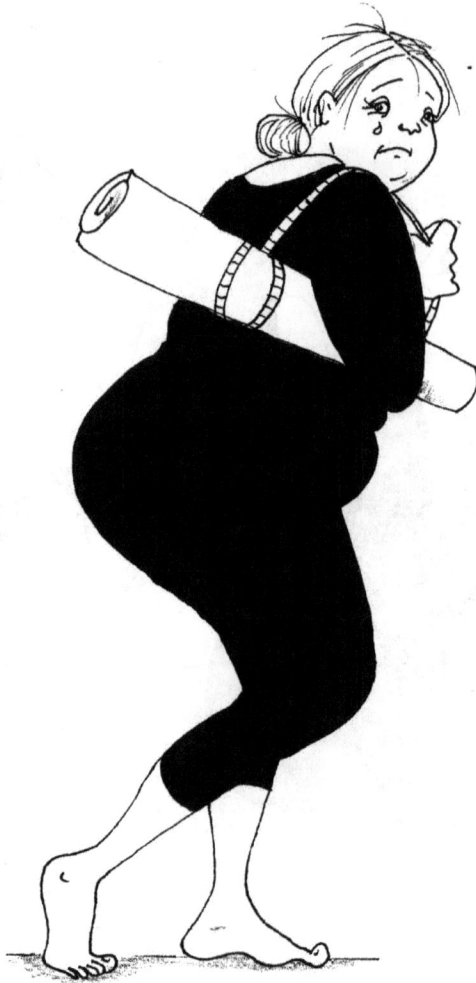

She picked her things up off the floor

And waddled meekly towards the door.

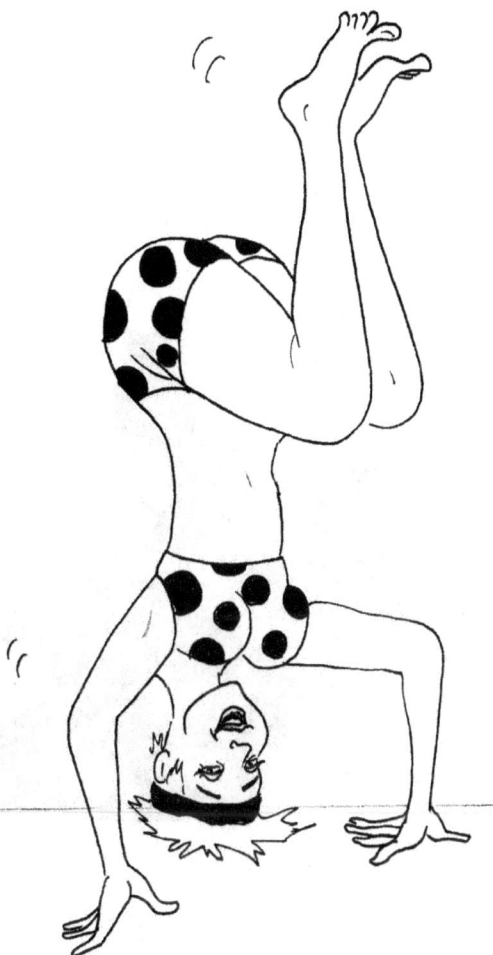

But just as she was almost out,

Across the room she heard a shout...

`Hey! Not so fast,´ the teacher said

Whilst upside down and on her head.

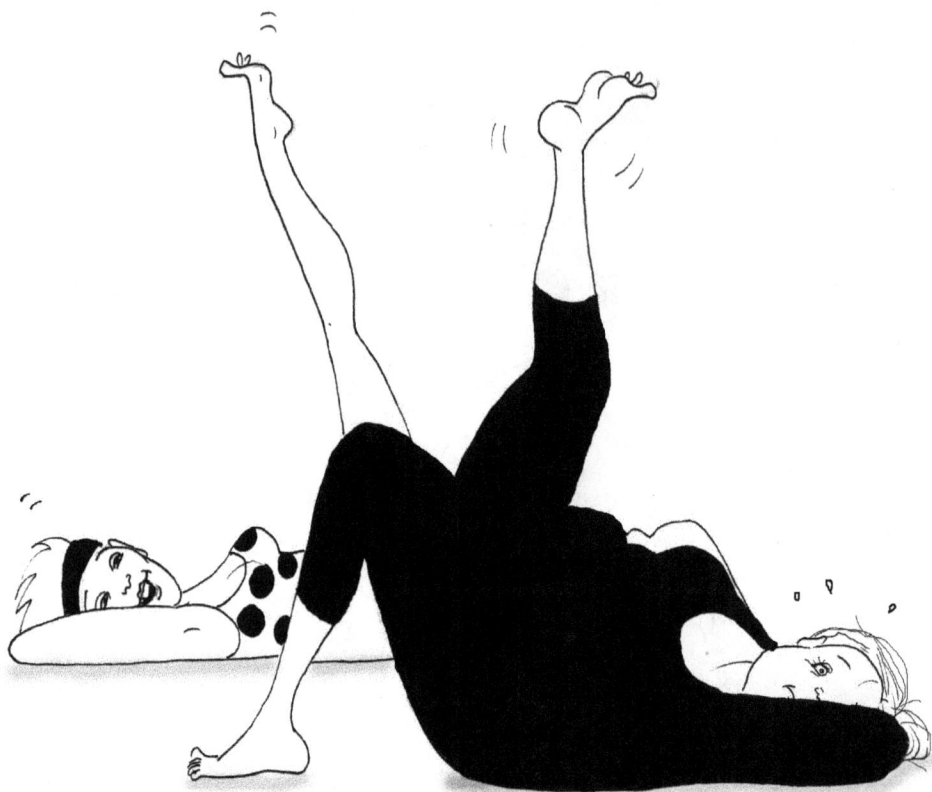

Don´t look so sad. It´s not so bad.

·I´ll show you what to do.

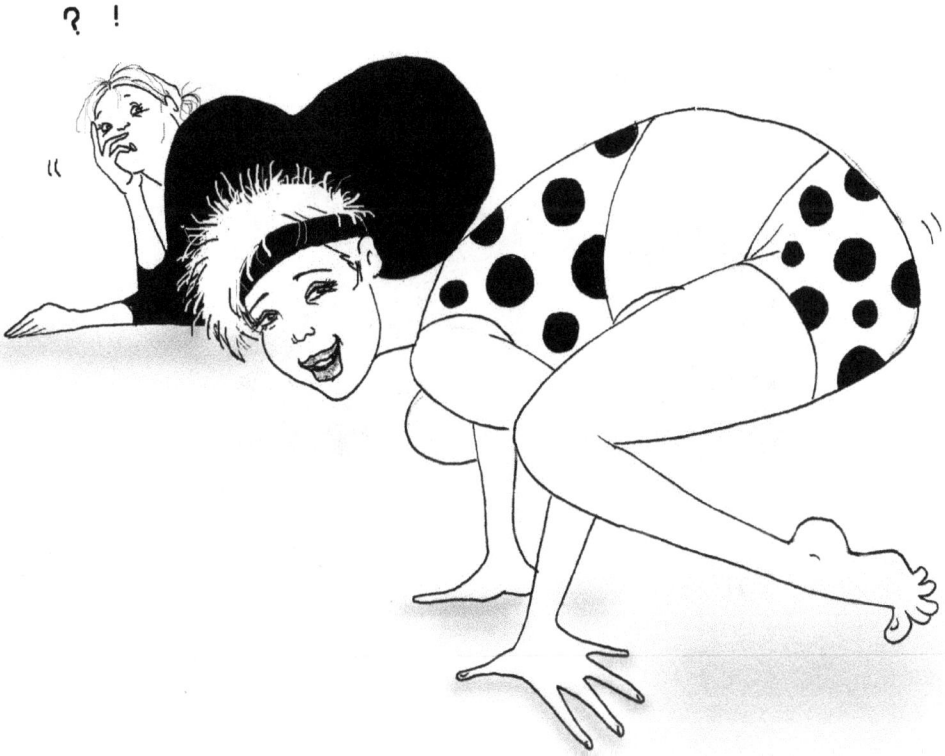

Move your body just like mine.

Hold your breath when I count two.

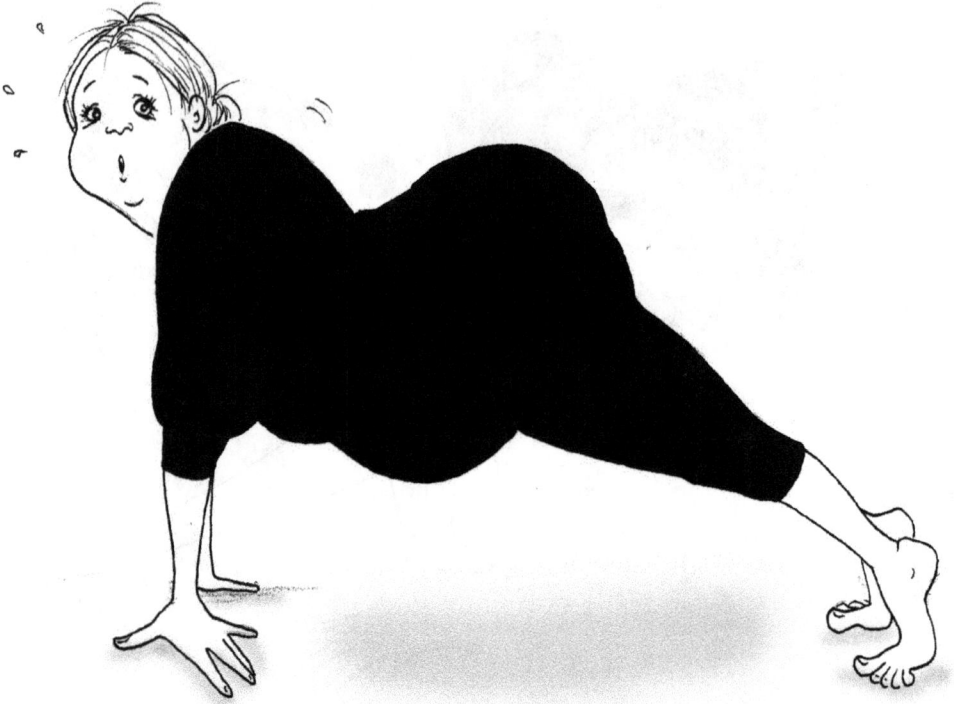

Close your nose. Breathe through your lips.

Squeeze in your tum and open hips.

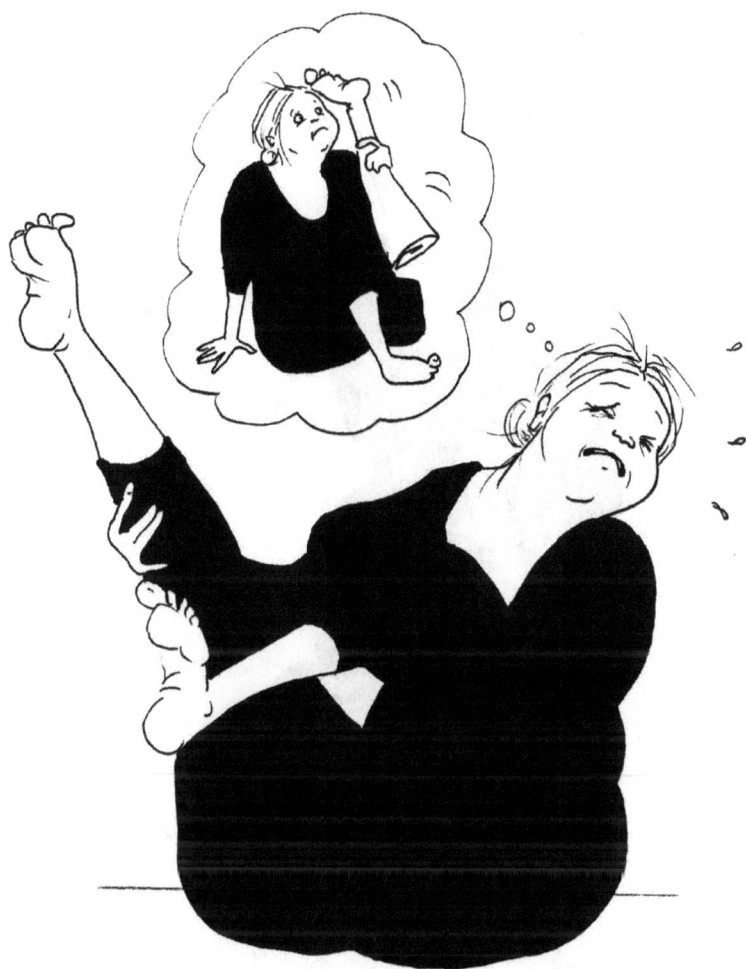

Unfold your ankles. Put them here.

Move that leg behind your ear.

`Are you kidding?´ Baba gasped.

`Surely not, while it´s attached?´

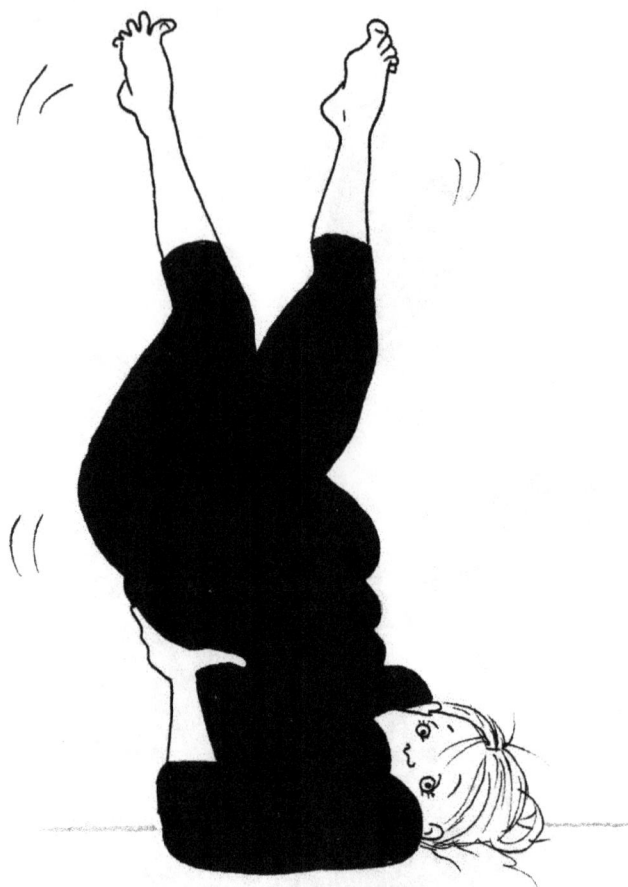

Inhale. Exhale. Feel your prana.

Before we do our next asana.

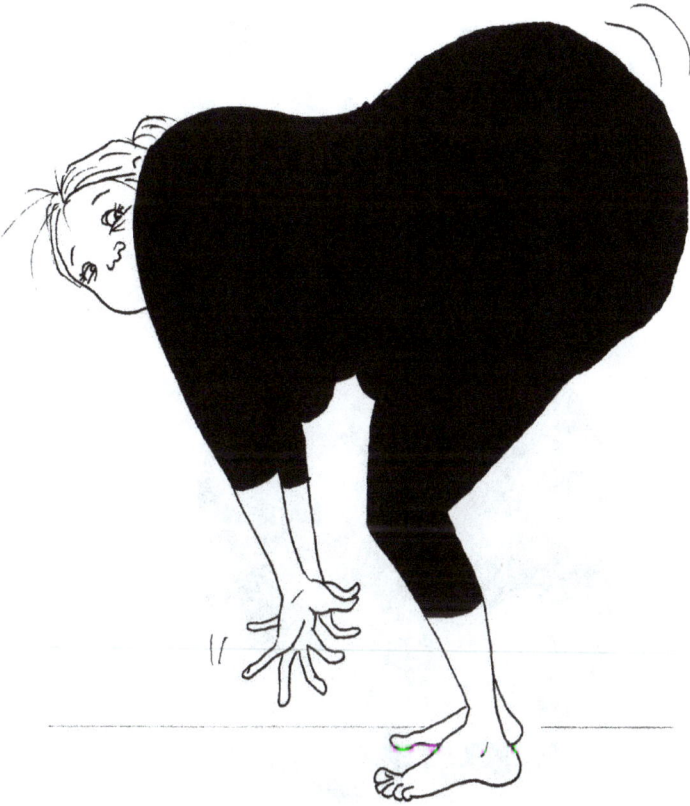

Stretch those bones

And reach your toes.

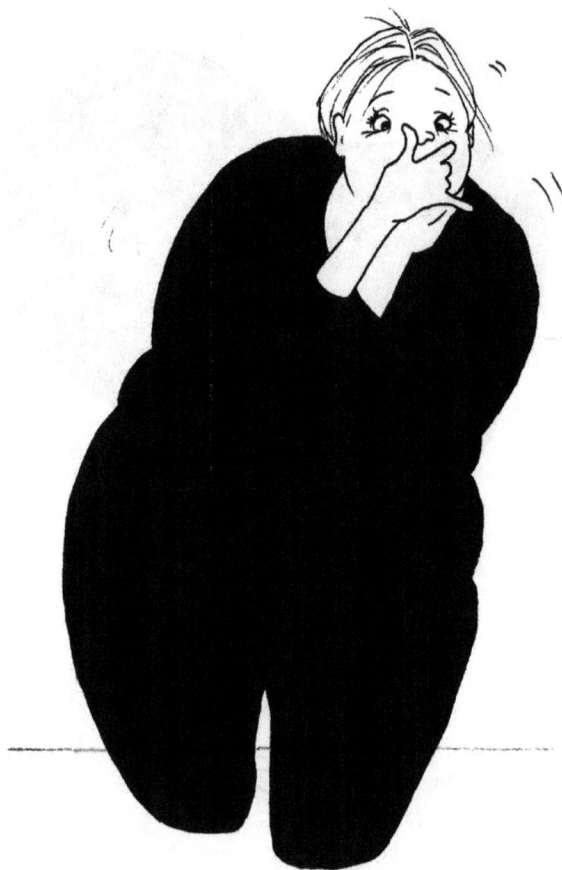

Bend that arm

With thumb on nose.

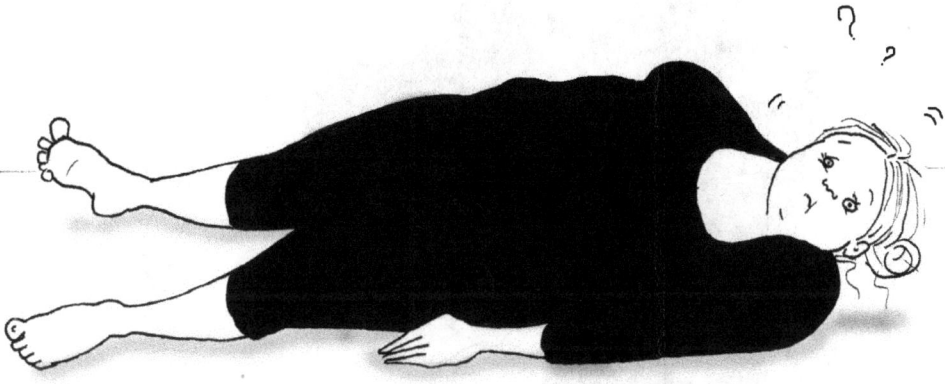

Now place your feet wide apart.

We're going to recap from the start.

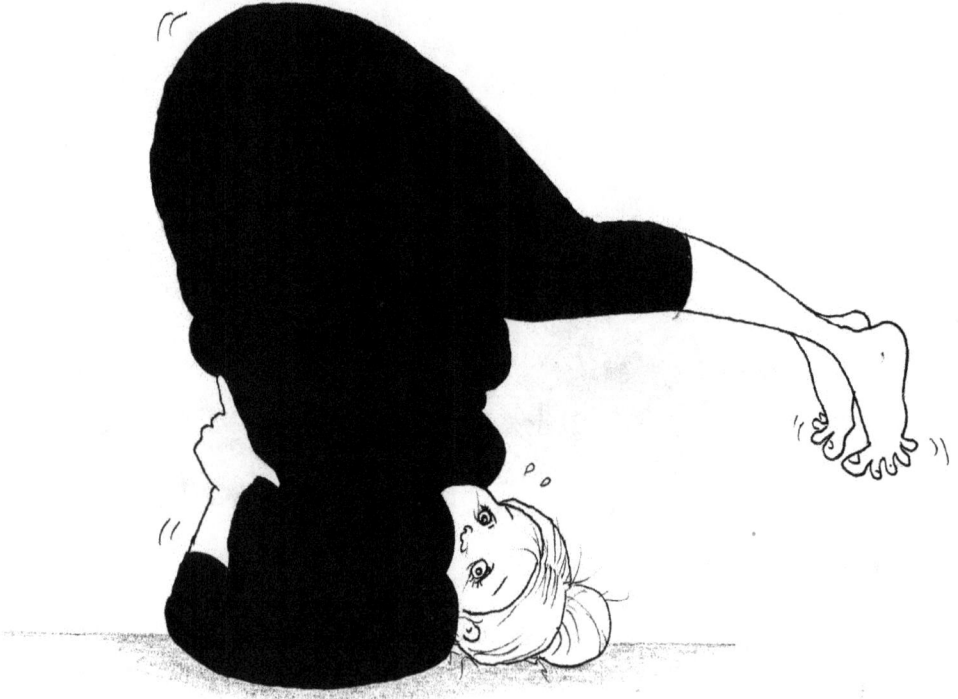

Baba did her best to fake it.

Fearing that she wouldn't make it.

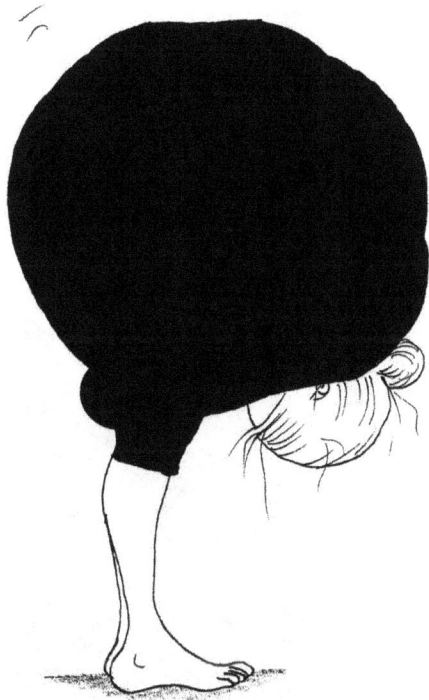

She took a breath,

Let out a sigh

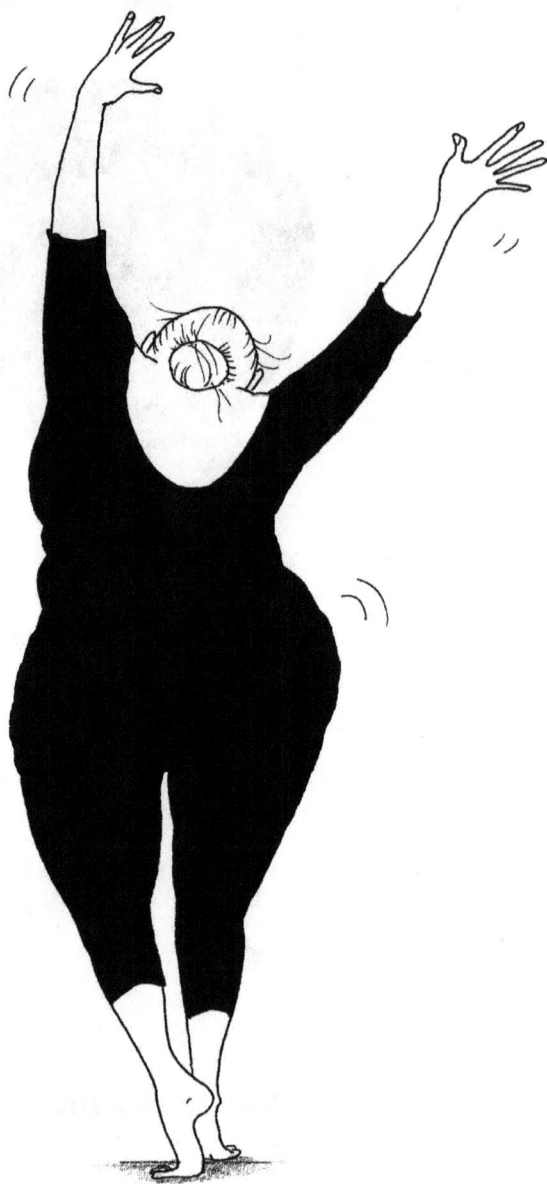

Then stretched her arms

Out way up high.

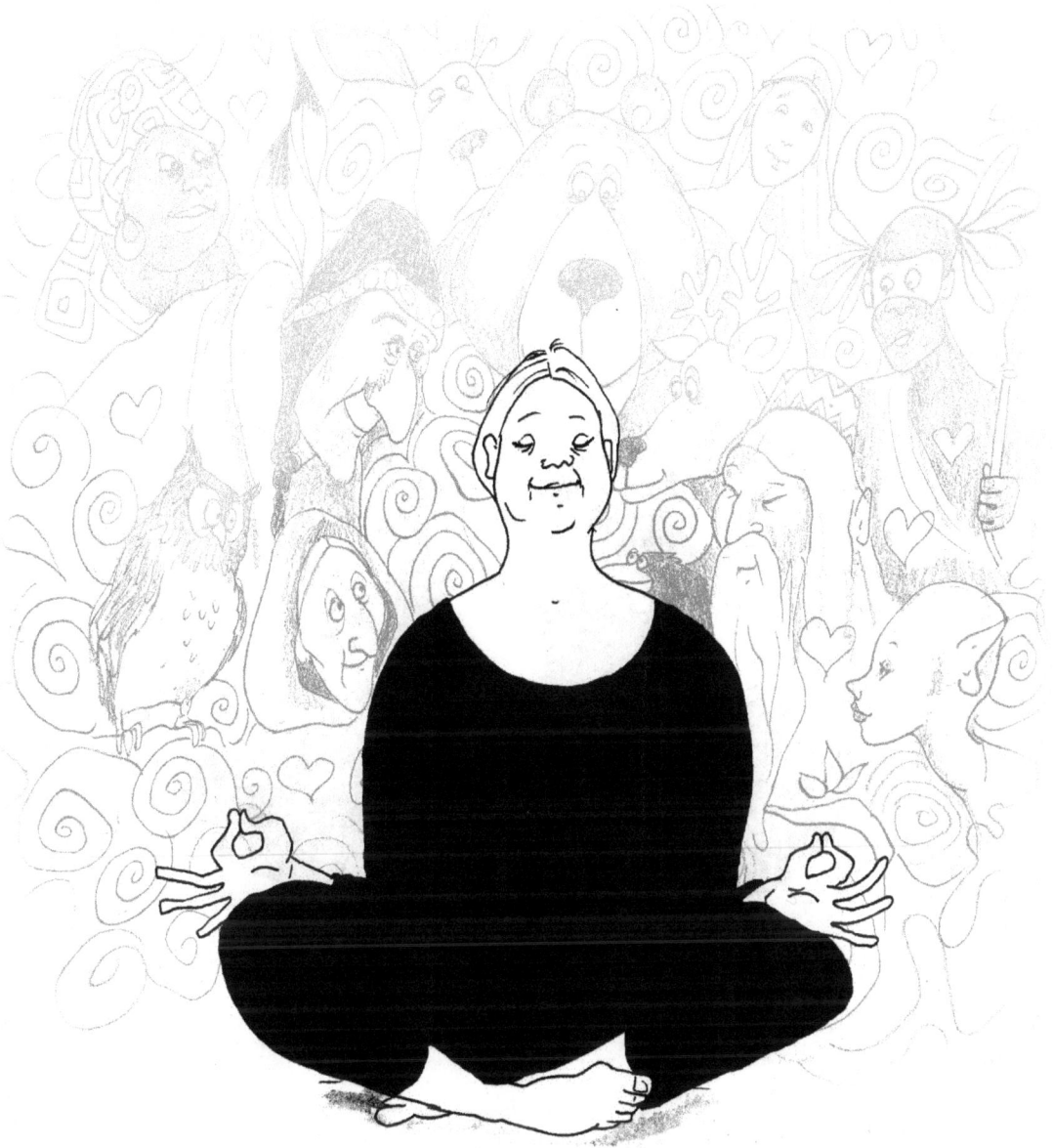

She closed her eyes. Reached deep inside.

Got in touch with her inner guides.

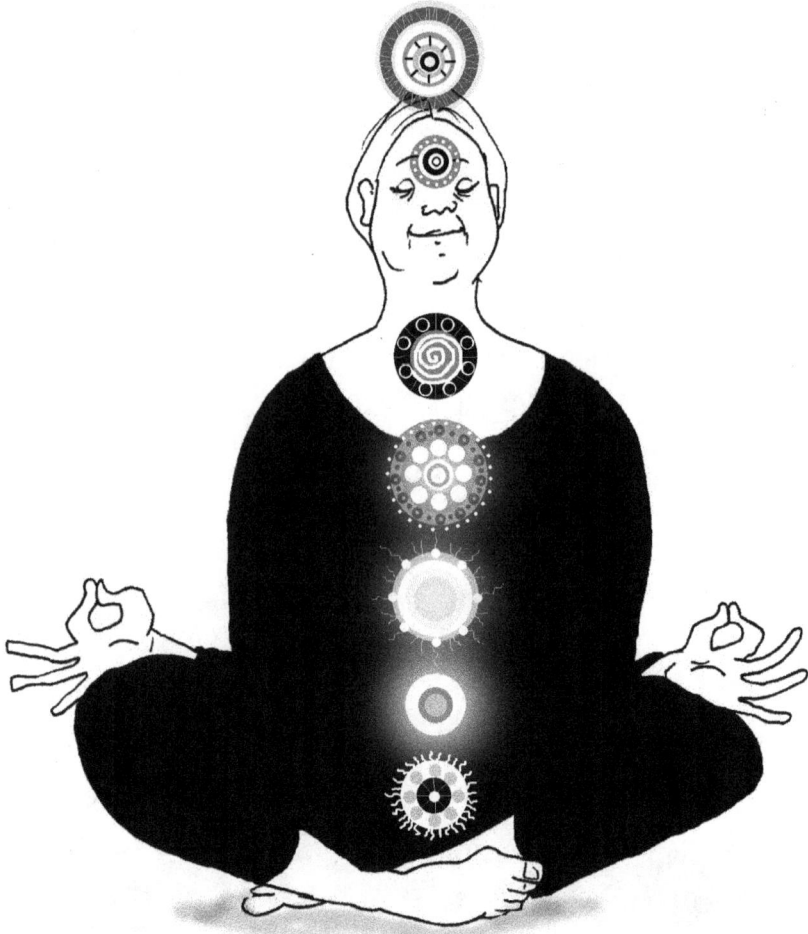

She freed her soul. She cleared her mind.

She felt her chakras all alligned.

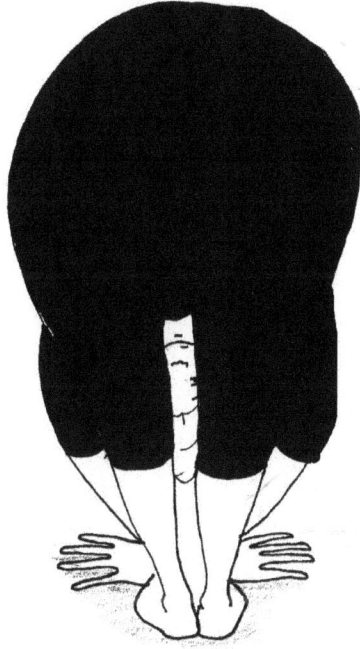

Feeling clear and quite elated.

She felt good and motivated.

She inhaled light. She exhaled deep.

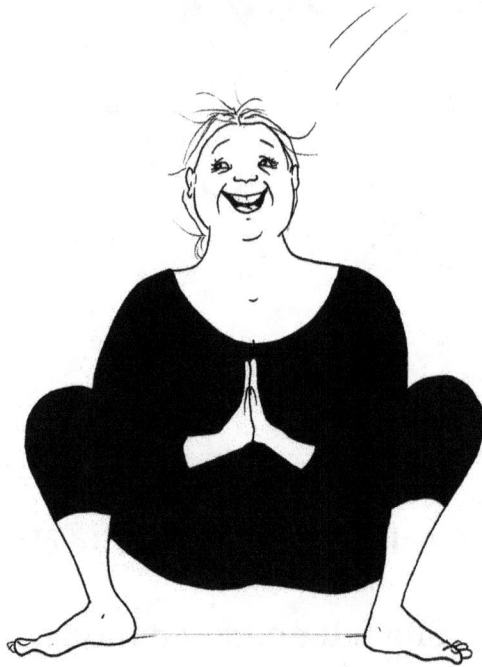

She did a squat.

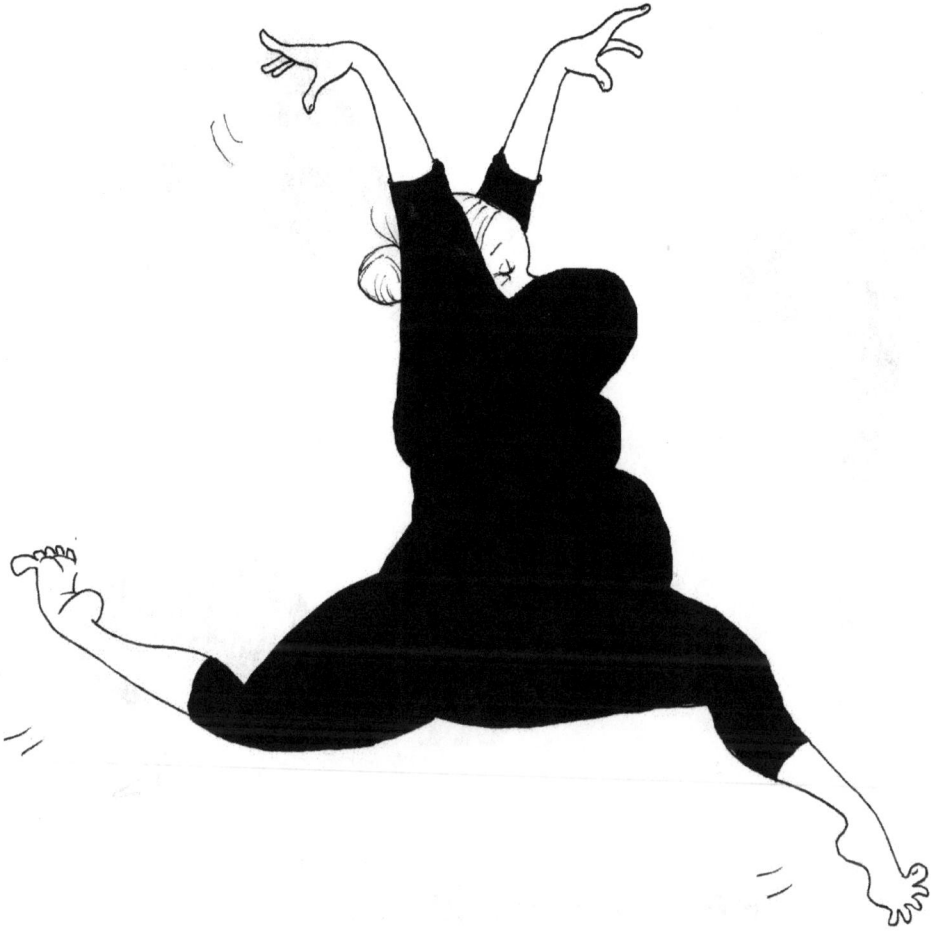

She did a leap.

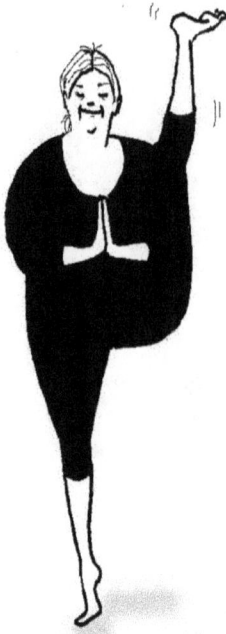

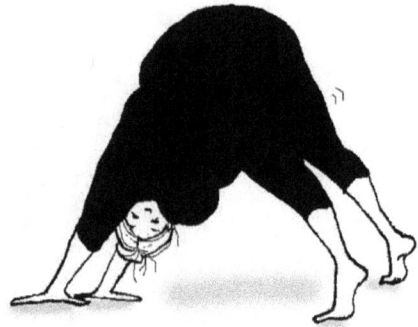

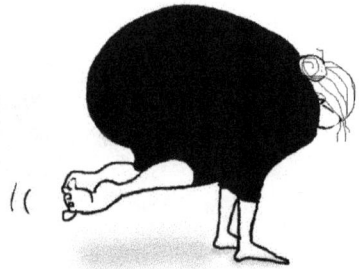

In front of all the others noses...

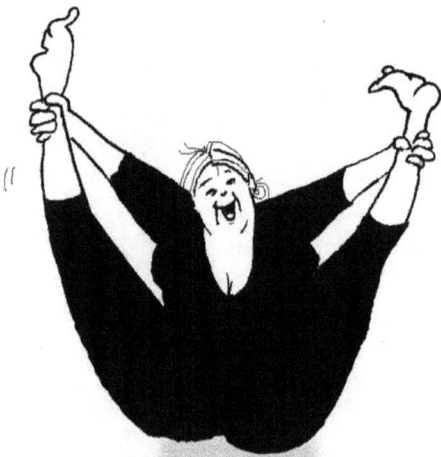

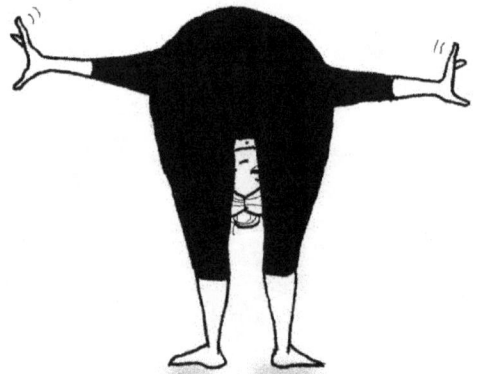

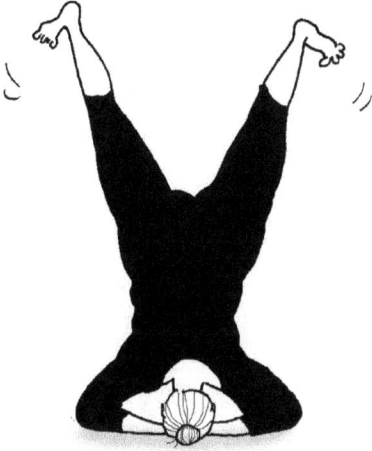

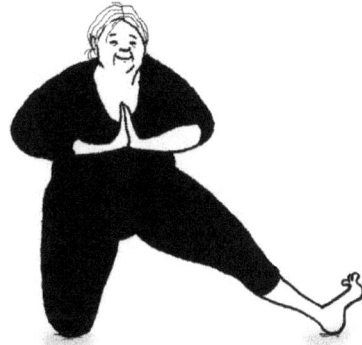

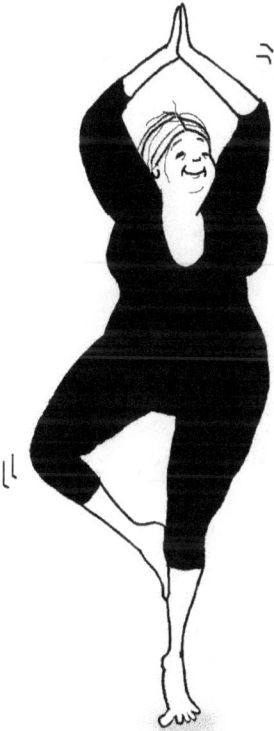

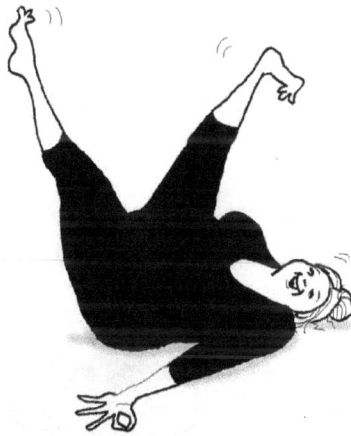

...She contorted into yoga poses.

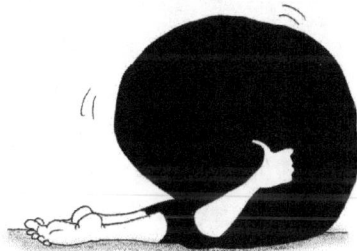

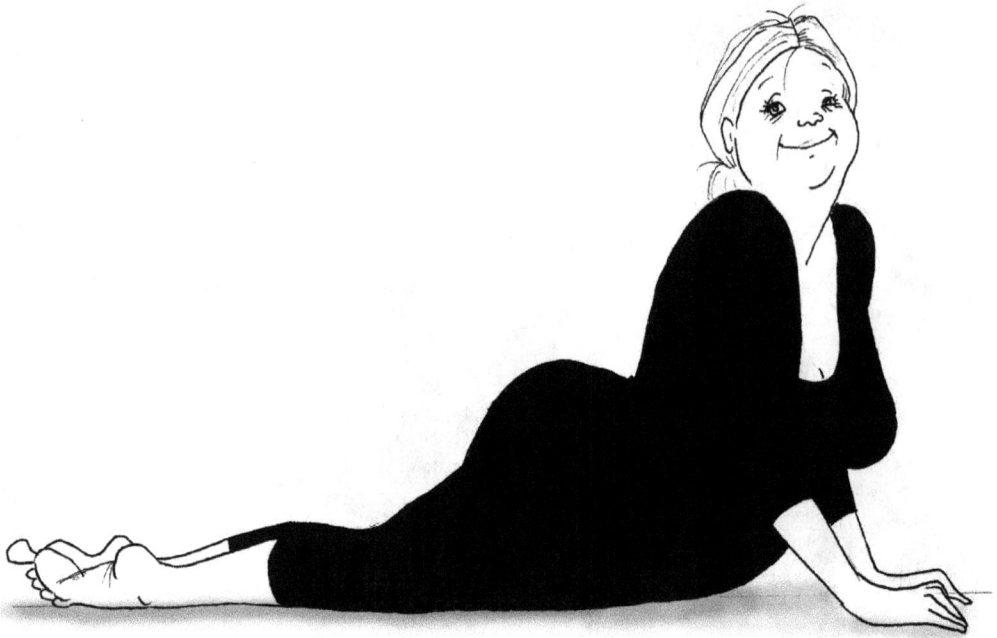

She did the Cobra.

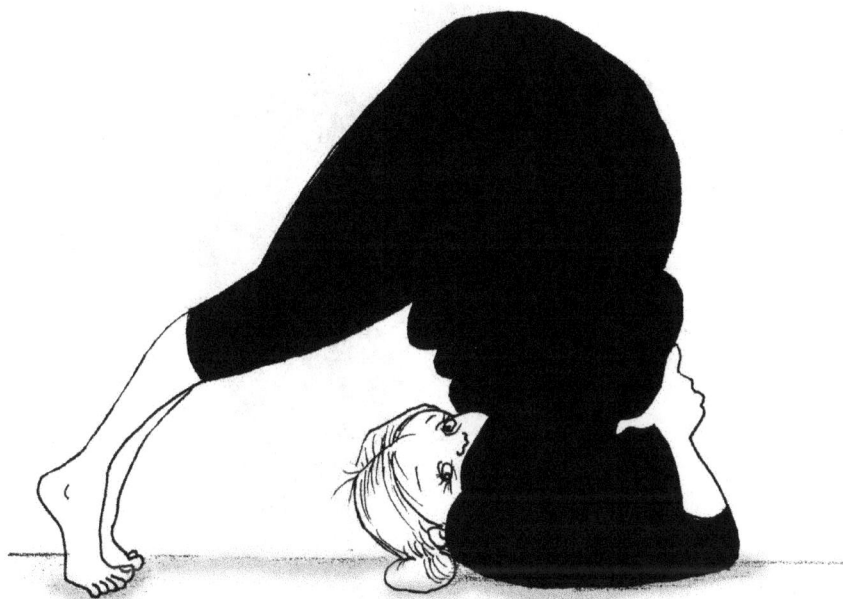

She did the Pough.

Totally present and in the Now.

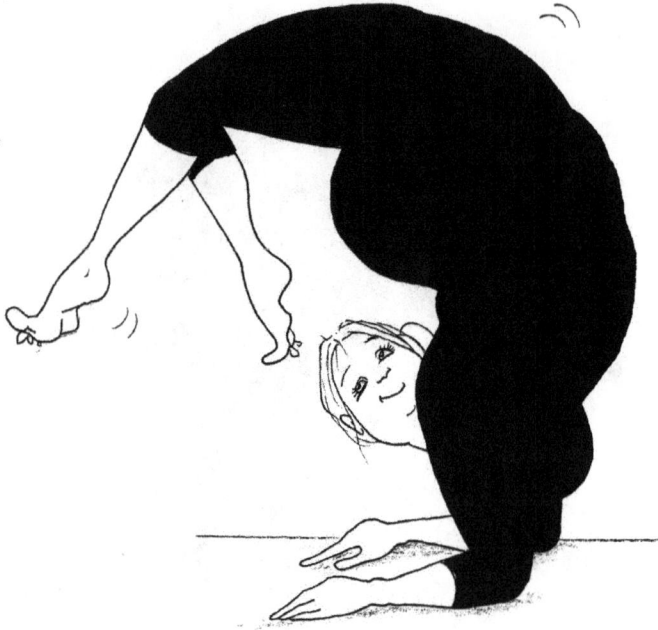

And like a french accordion,

She even did the Scorpion.

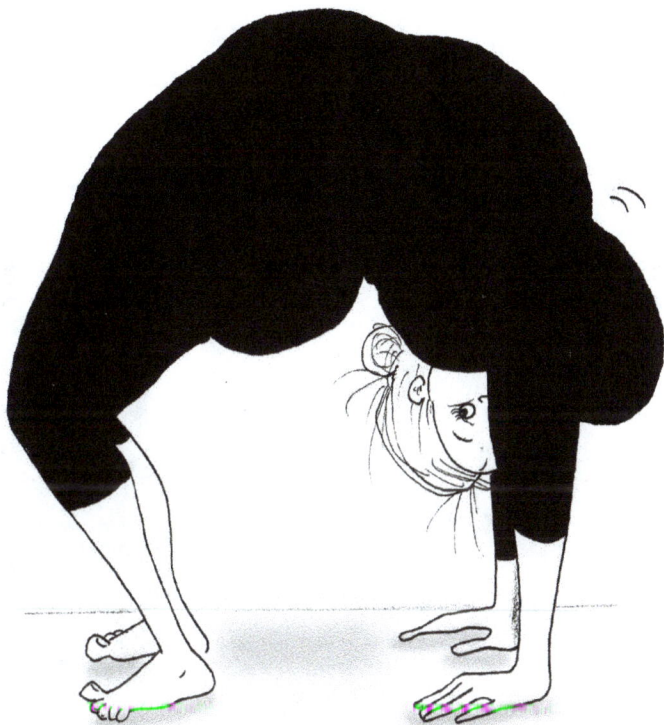

Just as class was ´bout to end.

Baba did a backward bend.

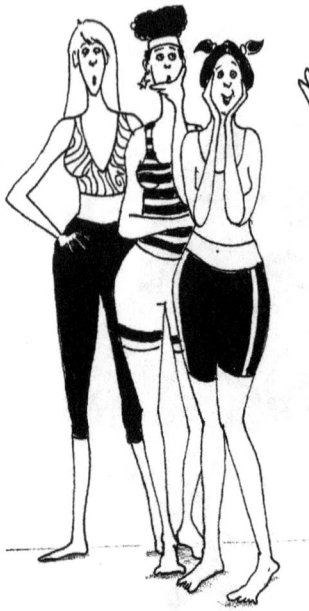

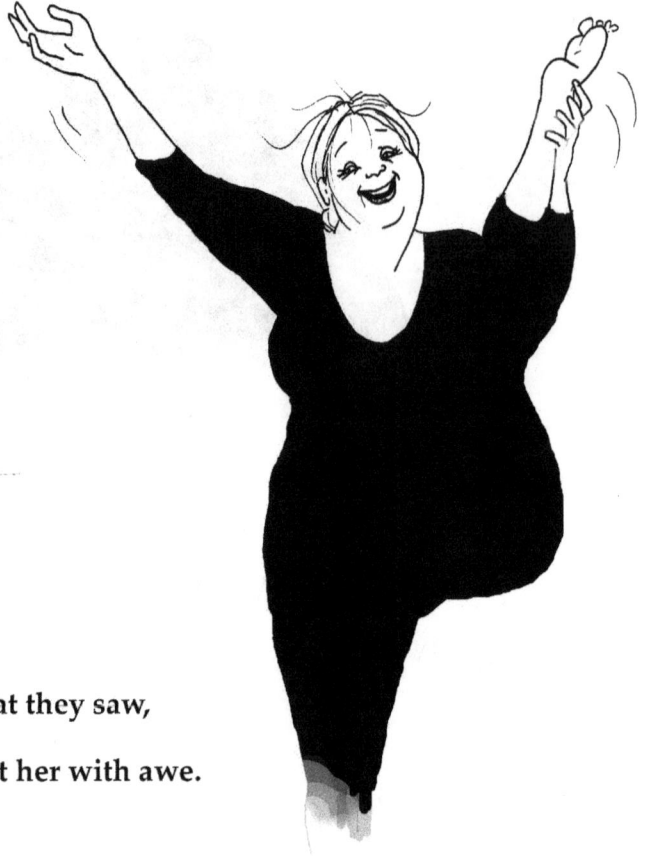

Hardly believing what they saw,

Her classmates looked at her with awe.

`You were great. We´re so impressed.

Please stay with us. You passed the test.´

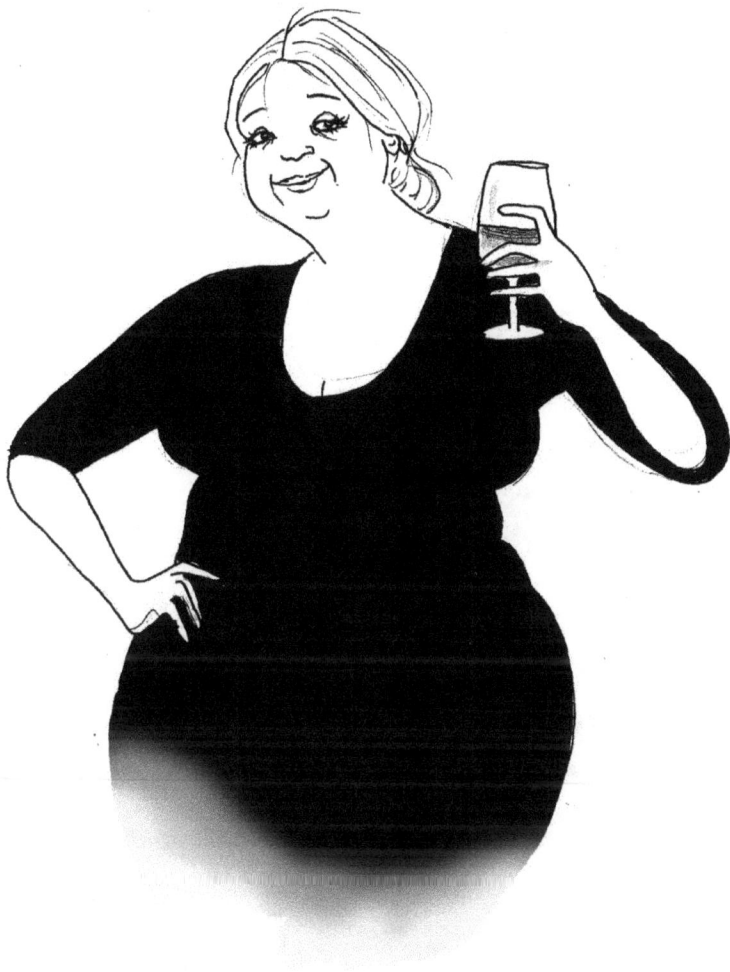

`Thank you, but I must decline.

I´d rather have a glass of wine.

So now I bid you Namaste,

And wish you all a lovely day.´

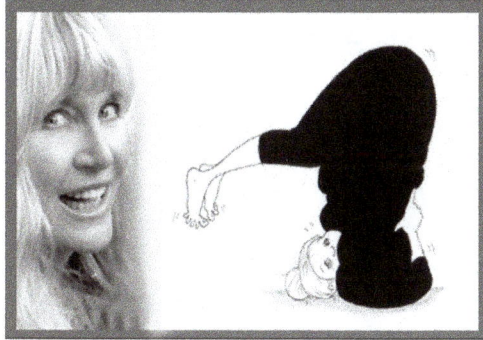

About Jakki

As well as an author, Jakki is an artist, illustrator and animator. She rarely goes anywhere without her sketchbook. She is passionate about using her art and humour to help address issues that need to be looked at more closely.

Jakki stumbled upon yoga many years ago when it was relatively unknown in the West. In those days, it was considered something weird and mysterious that came from India and that hippies did it. Fascinated by this ancient practice, she even managed to pick up a yoga teaching certificate and acquire a Hindi spiritual name.

Greatly inspired and determined to remind everyone (but mostly herself) that yoga is for everyone, she wrote and illustrated `Baba goes to Yoga.´

For all the teachers who have crossed my path so far.

For those who have passed on to other realms. For those

that are still living and for those I have yet to meet.

My teachers come to me in many forms; as relatives,

as friends, as strangers, as animals and as challengers.

I have much to learn. I am grateful.

Namaste

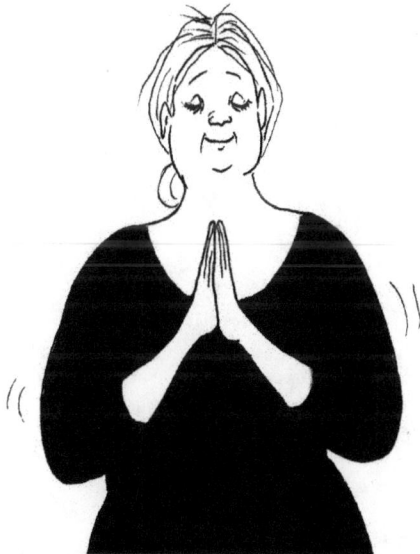

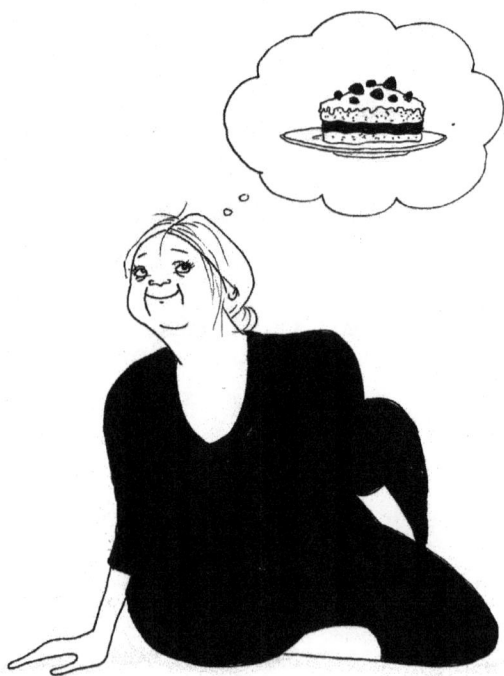

www.ingramcontent.com/pod-product-compliance
Lightning Source LLC
Chambersburg PA
CBHW051348290326
41933CB00042B/3329

9780956410825